My Pain Runs Deep

...But My Purpose Runs Deeper

Poetic Pain

I get lost deep in my thoughts
My mind draws a blank
What next? The little voice says
Now it's time to think
Not think but free write
Let it all out
No holding back
Even the loudest shout
I scream so loud
But not physically
On paper I had to release it
The inhale that had been waiting
Long hours to be set free
The time was now
And the person was me
The emotions I endure daily
Builds up from pain testing my patience
No more trying to fake it
I'm in my mind like I can't take it
but this poetic pain
I must sustain
It eases my mind
Like the gentle rain
And calms my soul
Now I'm back in control
Only until the next episode...

I...

Carry this pain with purpose
Yes, it's all worth it
You left me all alone
Cold inside my feelings so far gone
I'm stuck and numb
Why you? How come?
Permanently damaged
But everyday I'm healing
What am I doing?
Simply just dealing
Trying to make a way
What really happened?
I'd rather not say
One bad event
Now I'm left reminiscing
Finding ways to cope
Living in high hope
That one day you'll return
But for now, we live and learn
That until next time
.... will be okay

Your Faith

It's crazy how hard times test you
For situations to become a breakthrough
It becomes difficult to believe
That you will ever succeed
You become numb and eager
But your faith it gets deeper
When visions can be misleading
The outcomes are quite intriguing
Never second guess
What could be your greatest test
Because one wrong action
Can make your faith start lacking

Mistakes

Be careful of those mistakes
The ones you double make
The ones by choice
No matter the voice
The ones you try to escape
Never get too caught up
Because your feelings could erupt
Leaving you stuck in time
Many thoughts running through your mind
Now you are left thinking
Did you mess up completely?
Or could you turn the situation around?
Flip that frown upside down?
Double back and take real action
No matter what you face
The time is now
There is no race
Just fix your silly mistakes

Emotionally scarred

I found a love I never want to lose
I found a love I never want abused
I found a love so real and true
A love you thought came right from you
But this love oh so brand new
Has made my sky once again blue
Has brought on a clearer view
Has tightened all my loose screws
I found a love I used to refuse
A love I once put on snooze
So now if I had to choose
The love I found can't be renewed
Because the love I found doesn't come in twos
The love you expressed only left a bruise
And even left me so confused
The love you showed came with funny clues
Ones I tried to simply excuse
Because the love you gave had bad reviews
The new love I found is permanently tattooed

Am I asking too much?

It won't be easy
So, I'll get right into it
Are you ready for this?
More importantly are you prepared for this?
Can you put your pride aside for me?
And go places we can never forget?
Can you treat my heart like it hasn't been shattered?
Make my past seem like it never happened?
Can you help me discover new beginnings?
Give me the best intrigued feeling?
Or am I asking too much?
Accept me as I am flaws and all?
Pick up the phone for every single call?
Promise to never leave me nor stray away?
As we agree to take this love thing day by day.
Be the one to brighten up my smile?
And vow to give me the best years worthwhile?
Or am I asking too much?
One day I pray to get what's best
Doing things I wouldn't have to regret
To find my person and be set free
And I'm most certain
That now it's you and me
So, if I haven't already asked too much
Can you be the one to give my heart that adrenaline rush?

Baby Would You?

I know it's new to you
But I just want the real truth:
If I'm falling for you too fast
Baby would you catch me?
If I'm hanging on by threads
Baby would you untangle me?
If I lose you on the path
Baby would you come find me?
It's as simple as little things like that
So many questions I can ask
But baby are you willing?
So many things we can endure
But is it worth revealing?
Too many times I had to ask
So, I'm not risking
To be with you and deal with you
Before the feelings
If I'm a mess and you don't know why
Baby would you still stick around?
Between the lows and the highs
Baby would you still hold it down?
If I'm too caught up with pride
Baby would you still let me drown?
Insecurities winning with exposure
While these mixed emotions pass over
I just want you so much closer
Until I regain my composure
Baby would you promise to ride this rollercoaster?

Deep

I held you so close
For so long
Not knowing if I could escape
The four walls you had me trapped in
Calling it love
But was it really?
Had me so far gone
Feelings way in too deep
I would cry so loud
But only my thoughts could hear me
So caught up in your life
That I almost lost myself
A prisoner I no longer was
For the path that I left

How Could You?

You made those promises
Made it sound all good
Never was straight honest
You fed yourself lies
Trying to protect everyone else
Making excuses for their actions
Always neglected yourself
Until the point when nothing was left
You ran your well dry
And now all I ask is why?
I'm over it
I'm so through
One last question though,
How could you?

Why Me?

Sometimes it's bad to question
But you left me second guessing
It was my patience you were always testing
And my heart you kept racing
I'm sick and tired of the games
When were you going to change your ways?
Maybe we could have worked it out
But too many times I had to shout
Why me?

Becoming

Some like to keep up with the past me
But that's because they no longer have access
Going down the road of who I used to be
As if they can't seem to get pass that
It wasn't easy making a change
Dealt with some inner issues I had to rearrange
My flaws, my rules, my goals
So much had to be altered
For the life I chose

Misery Loves Company

My emotions get mixed up with my actions
When those friends left, I thought it was something I lacked in
Thinking I wasn't enough
When in reality, I must have been too much
Misery loves company and they were deceitful
Things they would do left me saying "I can't believe you"
Actions never matched their words
Too many occasions I was unheard
Unknown conversations of hate
Often ignored due to energy I refused to reciprocate
Misery loves company but I insisted on happiness
It demanded rages of anger, but I wasn't having it

Her Soul Cry

Her smile was so fake
You know, the one she wore on her face
Because her composure would say otherwise
Due to the drained look in her eyes
She would stare in the mirror
And often ask herself questions
Ones that often had her second guessing
She was craving things and I'm not talking food
I'm talking things that would put her in a bad mood
Her soul cried out
But she wouldn't listen
So, she began to pout
And eventually went back missing

Trust Issues

It became hard to love
And harder to open up
Not knowing who to trust
Kept my feelings bottled up
So many questions revolving
Who can I count on?
Is this a set up?
Why me?
Are these real feelings?
All the different I miss you's
Were the reasons for my trust issues

What I Been Through

If I told you only half
You wouldn't believe it
Because the smile I wear
Some misread it
Sometimes I'm actually happy
Other times I'm hiding pain
Actual pain nobody cared about
Until I disappeared again
But then the pain got too heavy
And now people noticed
It wasn't just coping
Every angle, every view
Was what I had been through

How would You Feel?

Tell me something:
If it happened to you,
What would you do?
Same shit you put me through
You wouldn't be able to handle it
I was cautious with your feelings
But you were careless with mine
How could you be so selfish with time?
I became fed up, I was disgusted
I could no longer fathom the disrespect
So, I did what was best for me
Ended something I thought I could build
And all I want to know is:
If it happened to you,
How would you feel?

It's My Life

Nobody can change my mind
What's for me will always be mine
The route I chose
Even the long dark roads
Was what I knew would prepare me
Molded me into who I am today
Many things some won't approve of
Simply because I chose to rise above
I'm not better than anybody
I'm bigger than the situation
I choose me now and not population
Because It's my life

I'm In Control

No matter what I do
No matter what they say
No matter the delays
I always get my way
I may not know how
I may not know when
I may not know why
But I know it's within
Some things take time
Others take work
But with my faith
I'll surely get what I deserve
I won't break
I won't fold
I'm built to stay
I remain in control

I overcame

Many loses I took
But each one was a lesson
Some bumpy roads I shook
And I call it all a blessing
Cause what you sent to break me
Only made me better
Made me stronger
Every storm I weathered
Trials and trials of pain
But thank God I overcame

Abandoned

Lost my identity going through pain alone
Sitting there wondering if the pain was gone
Drowning in the many tears I had to wipe away
Telling myself I would be okay
I spent hours in solitude
Only surrounded by the drenched tissues
It felt as though I was rejected
By people who I thought cared
Revealing how I was neglected
But in reality, my presence was really spared

Oh you in your Feelings Huh?

I let you have your way for a while
But when it was my turn there was no smile
You couldn't take what you dished out
And you knew it would hurt without a doubt
Stuck reminiscing in the past
The shit we had you wanted to last
So you say anyway
I knew my heart was where you played
Until I ended your silly games
See, I caught on to your lies and schemes
What was my reality was never in my dreams?
I knew I had to escape
Before I was raped
And no not physically but mentally
Because you had me stuck in lust
Releasing our bond was a definite must

Apologize

So many lonely nights
But, I blame myself
So many doors closed on me
As if I had nothing left
I had some inner healing to do
I let it get too deep
And I was lost with no clue
There were barely times I would sleep
How can I overcome this?
I asked
You would think I knew right?
Wrong! because it wouldn't have got this bad
It was bad to where I felt it
And I mean hard
My words, my actions, most importantly my heart
From the beginning to the middle and end
If you ever met me then,
You would say I was scarred
But I'm healing now
Thank God for deliverance
What was sent to break me
Turned into bravery
I had to rediscover my purpose
Find myself and reveal
I look in the mirror
And it was so much I realized
But to sum it all up
I simply apologized

Fed up

I was sick of the lies
And grew tired of the hatred
So much to hold in
There was no way I could fake it
Too much at once
Why me one would ask
Then there was me
I desired change from my past
I couldn't keep on living the same
Somehow it was still me I blamed
Until I became fed up

A drought on love

Was it my feelings?
Was it my actions?
Did I not make enough happen?
Didn't know where to turn
Didn't know when I would learn
I just knew it wasn't lasting
So much for happily ever after's
To some love never mattered
It became distant
Disappearing more day by day
Thinking I could fix it
The heartaches would replay
Sweat tears and even some blood
One would declare
There was a drought on love

Weathered Storm

When they took you
I thought I was through
I thought my life was over
No way I could hold my composer
No way its true
This can't be you
I'm facing reality
But still in denial
It broke me down
Deep down to my lowest
But that was then
And this is now
I used to sit and ask Why me
But now I say Try me
I was built for the storm
Nobody thought I would ever weather
My dear brother is gone
But this journey is my greatest endeavor

I Choose My Happiness

I used to put others first
You know, trying to keep everyone happy
Sudden rages of hateful outbursts
I became one that was very snappy
I disliked feeling like this
I knew something had to quickly give
I had to make some sacrifices
For the life I wanted to live
So, I started to choose me
Then I began to see
What I wanted for so long
Some could care less
But I felt so strong
Because I finally chose my happiness

Where the Love at?

Said you was with me, but you lied
Too many times I sat and cried
Sitting there wondering why
And if I should put my feelings aside
Now I'm wondering where the love at.

Too many things you needed to know
But it was times you didn't show
So, each time I had to go
And then my tolerance had got too low
Now I'm seeing where the love at!

If it's a love that's there
It's not for me, I'm aware
Because you left me with this blank stare
As you clearly showed me you didn't care
And it finally revealed where the love was at

Settling

In life I thought I was chasing a dream
But getting older, it seemed as if that dream was chasing me
Moving further and further away from my goals
Really made it look like I was no longer in control
The life I was living was no longer mine
Going with the flow just existing with time
I made mistakes, I took some Ls
I had some wins and even some fails
But again, this wasn't what I imagined
Sometimes most things just were happening
I no longer felt ambitious
My creativity bar was low
Going through stages though I wouldn't admit this
Even though my actions begin to reflect and show
Bare minimum and not even a second thought
Was the only effort I put forth instead of what I was taught
I began to do a lot of questioning
Because my life was no longer leveling
It just seemed as if I was settling

No More Cloudy Days

The sun will shine again
And when it does, you'll be there
Due for a win
Because life can seem unfair
We become numb to living
In this world with some people missing
But life must continue
All the joy you need is within you
The cloudy days are going away
It's time to shine and seize the day

Can we talk?

Hold on, wait a minute
It's some things we never finished
So now that I got your attention
I'm just wondering if we could fix it

It's a lot I want to say
But I know emotions will get in the way
So, before you begin to play
Can you just be serious for today?

So much on my mind
And I feel we're running out of time
Because my peace I'm trying to find
But it's like you're not trying to rewind

The bad days I want to erase
But it seems you want to retrace
And I'm just trying to escape
The memories I look to as a disgrace

Your actions leave me with confusion
Some may even call me stupid
Because your love for me has been proven
Now I'm searching for a solution

Anxious

Randomly I get this feeling
My throat closes
My skin is flushed
My heart starts racing
Yet I'm in no rush
My thoughts run wild
My mind draws blank
I can't breathe yet I'm awake
This feeling I get
Comes and goes
What is going on?
Most won't know
It's called a panic attack
And when it comes my energy lacks
It's like I get knocked off track
Patiently waiting on my body to bounce back

Colliding Thoughts

Quite often we experience the unexpected
And sometimes our thoughts feel quite neglected
But when we sit and wonder what's to come next
Our thoughts often collide and become hectic
It's like our intuition feeds off confirmation
But what the eyes see are most times hallucinations
We can never agree on what is real
Which leads us right into a big ordeal
These thoughts they drive us completely insane
From one situation to another it wrecks our brain
Yet somehow, we manage to survive it all
Colliding thoughts are not your final call

Confessions

There's a truth in these confessions
And I won't leave anyone guessing
But the way I been feeling
Has been quite revealing
Not sure if you noticed
But I haven't been focused
Haven't been showing up
Times had really gotten rough
Felt as if I was all alone
Especially in the comfort of my home
My feelings would get the best of me
Canceling plans was a guarantee
Just not up for being on the scene
Sticking to my same routine
Praying for better days to happen
Waiting to live a better life I had imagined
See adversity would visit me quite too often
Now I proceed to live with caution
I'm aware of my surroundings
Aware of my friends
Aware of my actions
Aware of my health
And so much more
But most importantly
Being more aware than ever before

Desires

I want to be a delicate individual
One who doesn't have to put up a wall
The kind of female who isn't on a fight or flight risk
But ready to risk it all
I've given some of my best years of love
To some of the worst kind of people
But I live with no regrets
And certainly, no wishes of evil
I desire a prayed for love
A love I don't have to question
A love that won't leave me second guessing
I want the small gestures that include effort
And not the small arguments that make my head hurt
I want to be able to say I prayed for this
And know that we are both able to fully commit
I want to be your sunshine through a storm
And love you in any form
Your high when you feel low
That way you know I'm never letting go
I want a prayed love that people admire
Yes, these are my simple desires

Bear With Me

Be patient with my heart, it's a little fragile
Be patient with my love, it's all shattered
Be patient with my tears because they matter
Be patient with my actions, they become a battle
Be patient with my thoughts, they tend to scatter
Be patient with my journey, it's written in chapters
Be patient with my jokes, it's only for laughter
Be patient with my pace, in case you move a little faster
Be patient with my personality, I am no actor
Be patient with my life, in case it becomes a disaster

 I say all of this to say that I am not perfect
but if you stick around and bear with me
I'll show you why it's worth it

Prisoner of my thoughts

Headstrong I'm in the game
Yet I feel so alone
Is my mind playing tricks?
I'm feeling a little cloned
So many words I want to utter
But my mouth, it barely murmurs
And even if I could, I'd probably stutter
About my mind that often wonders
It's a simple game I often play
I sometimes wonder who can relate
It seems like I'm not moving fast
My mind however is doing the dash
I got to find out how to escape
I know that there is some way
It's a blessing being me
Now all I want is my mind to be set free

Naked

Clothed in scars and bruises
I don't think I'll ever be pretty
Layered with emotions and feelings
Because so many betrayed me
How can I be loved with all this baggage?
Some may see and label me as damaged
It's like the more I try and open up
The higher my protective wall builds
Trying to protect my peace, my feelings erupt
Calming them down with writing skills
Naked of who I'm used to being
At the sight of comfort, I'm usually fleeing
Healing is what I want
But sometimes I act nonchalant
Because I'm scared to let my guard down
But I know my wardrobe will come around
So, until I can enjoy my naked
You get to see what trauma created

The Great Escape

Lost deep in my thoughts
Not knowing if I'll be found
Some treasured faults
Left lying around
Not kept on purpose
Just wanted to know if the situation was worth it
I had a share of lessons to learn
In my years I've been burned
And in some cases, easily provoked
Mainly by people I cared about the most
So, inside my head is where I live
For now, until I can learn to forgive
No more trying to hide and runway
It's time to plan my great escape
There is a beautiful world awaiting me
It's my time now to be set free
Free from all the trauma and pain
Writing for me feels like dancing in the rain
My passion is my great escape

I am she

What a beautiful soul
Yet so damaged and hurt
She played a huge roll
In showing up first
Being there for everyone
Except herself
Now she is the one who needs the help
On the edge of defeat
She holds it together
Even during adversity
At the rise of another storm, she is ready to weather
From the outside looking in she's pretty
But so torn down inside
Not too many could really see
She was trying to swallow her pride
She had given up on allowing people close
Didn't want to have high hopes
Gave so much to ones not deserving
And always ended up being the one hurting
It's time to put an end to all that
And show everyone how she can bounce back

The Bigger Picture

It's not about what happened in the past
What I learned is most good things don't last
Can't reminisce about what went on
I know I must continue to push and be strong
Some things happen for specific reasons
And some people come and go based on seasons
We get to learn life lessons in the midst
All while trying to take big risks
There is so much more than people and places
But no matter what don't get complacent
The life we live is based on us
And living it to the fullest is a definite must
The future is always in our hands
So, when life throws you big demands
Just make sure you're ready
The journey will never be steady
Always remember the bigger picture

What Next?

Tragedy happens and then we wonder
What's next?
Where do we go from here?
How can we move on?
But there is hope in that tragedy
See my tragedy birthed a testimony
And you're currently reading part of it
No matter what you endure
When you heal put your heart in it
I thought I would never smile again
And now I smile as much as I can
Because I believed in me
My heart is finally being set free
Free from pain and misery
Because I lost a part of me

How Long?

How long do you sit and suffer in silence?
How long before you are completely quiet?
How long until you have no fight left?
How long before you begin to live with regrets?
How long before you see the real?
Then start to make a big ordeal
How long can it take to move on?
How long until the feelings are all gone?
How long until your big break?
How long until you realize how much you can take?
How long is too long before you finally digest the real life?

Shattered Life

As a growing woman
I've been through so much
Living with a fragile heart
Part of it filled with dust
Wondering where the love went
And why it became so hard to vent
Being betrayed by people close
Is part of what really hurts the most
Started losing people by the day
Never knowing what to say
All I have left is a bunch of puzzle pieces
But they consist of me and my life
Now I'm sitting here wondering
What is wrong and what is right
Slowly I'm putting the pieces together

Rise up Again

I take this pain and bottle it in
Release it with paper and pen
I hide so much behind a smile
Haven't been happy in a while
From grief to sorrow
I barely look forward to tomorrows
I can't stomach the empty feeling
I think it's time for some healing
Writing brings my confidence in
And speaking helps me rise again
I thank God for the gift placed in me
And when I release, I feel all free
It's something I take pride in
Each time I get to begin again

Born Again

You ever lose yourself so deep
That you forget who you really are
You ever cried so much
Until you've cried your eyes dry
You ever screamed so loud
Loud enough to make your voice hoarse
Those are real feelings of pain
Emotions getting the best of you
Those are feelings no one can explain
And they mostly happen out the blue
Sometimes we question why
And then receive no answers
Other times we wonder when things will change
Yet it's our life we must rearrange
We go into this very dark place
Not knowing how or when we will come out
It gets very lonely and boring
But we learn many lessons during this phase
A lot of things we must soak in
Before we come out and are born again

Slowly Fading Away

As our messages become distant
My feelings slowly fade away
Our face time no longer recent
And now I'm left with nothing to say
It's the way you act like everything is good
But then I express my emotions
And now I'm suddenly misunderstood
So, I go mute to keep down any commotion
You think that time is supposed to heal
Now you're MIA once again
Not knowing how I truly feel
For all your shenanigans I got to take in
As a female we go through a lot
And all we want is real genuine love
Too much I had to block
So now I'm trying to rise above
This time I'm putting me first
And I love how my happiness displays
I wouldn't say it was the worst
But everything I once felt faded away

The ReBirth

I knew I was different
But not many could see
There was something inside little ole me
Such powerful voice
But for so long it was trapped
Or was it sent away
And re-released by a trauma map
I had gone through so much
Half of it you wouldn't believe
Life hanging on by a crutch
Hoping a new one would be conceived
It was fear that almost had me
Until I realized my worth
I look back to the past and see
A different me had been rebirthed

Built for this

Be careful what you wish for
Things aren't always what they seem
What we think we have in store
Turns out nothing like the dream
Never to worry
No reason to fear
Despite the hurry
Breakthrough is near
Is it something you can handle?
Only time shall tell
Will it leave you burning like a candle?
Or full like the magical wishing well
Either way it's something you can't miss
Because you're built for this

Unlove You

I needed to unlove you
So that I could love myself
Because loving you
Was all I felt
I was so blinded by your actions
Nearly costing me my health
And your love was lacking
But you couldn't see
That I finally chose to focus on me
Unloving you was my best decision
Because being hurt was never in my vision

No Tears Left

Ever cried your eyes dry
So dry that it hurts to blink
Artificial tears you must apply
As you stand over a bathroom sink
So many tears shed
And you may be wondering why
Eyes bloodshot red
Under the impression that you're high
Pain and sorrow fill your life
Gutted with wounds
From the sharp edge of a knife
You become victim to abuse
From a pain you once excused

I Can't Help It

Protecting my energy at all costs
Because too many times I was taken advantage of
Lied to, stolen from, even verbally abused
Being nice for too long
Only left me healing from pain
Guarding my happiness and space
My discernment mind with the assist
I finally learned to put me first
Not 1 regret at all
The life I desire
Did not include neglecting me
So, when you see me truly happy
Just know I deserve it

Admiration

I love everything about you
Especially all that you do
It's the way you move with ambition
And the brown eyes that glisten
Look at how the hair flows with ease
That melanin gleaming in the sun is very easy to see
It's something about your facial expressions
That makes even your quietness a written book
They love to hear your articulated words
I guess that's why you write with passion
Can't forget about that beautiful smile
That makes every minute spent with you worthwhile

The Storm is Over

Too many dark nights
And not enough sunshine
Just when you think things are going right
One storm put's your whole life on the line
And when you think you've caught relief
Another incident leaves you full of grief
Smiling to hide the pain
That leaves your body and soul scarred
Dancing in the rain
Like you got a broken heart
As the grey skies clear
And you heal your wounds
Better days are near
For you to exit your cocoon

Change the Scenery

Vibes get old
People change
Loyalty is tested
What's real these days

Friends turn foe
Distance is outta range
Now life needs to be decompressed
For all the trauma that got in the way

A change of scenery is near
But only if desired
What some will fear
Most will soon require

A wind of fresh air
And calm soothing noises
An environment to share
With some positive voices

Free Yourself

We often wonder how many feels like us
Our words and mind get jumbled in a bunch
And we are left feeling numb and stuck
Now we are seeking who to trust
Because our mind tells us stick to our gut
It's time to get out of your head
No more living by what was said
Sometimes we tend to live on edge
But confine ourselves to limits
Knowing it could all change within a matter of minutes
It's time to enjoy life and free yourself

I Miss Me

It's the smiles that left
And the joy I felt
As the days pass by
I'm wondering why
It's me I miss

Or maybe it's the way I act
That makes look back
For the happiness I lack
Like damn it's me I miss

I'm quite sure I'm not alone
Pieces of me left when I was done wrong
Now I'm sitting here lost
And protecting my peace at all costs
Because it's me I miss

I miss me but she is not far
Sometimes we must rediscover who we are
Even if it takes a little while longer
We'll be making a comeback much stronger

Me Myself and I

When you feel all alone
Go look in the mirror
Such a beautiful soul
The image couldn't get much clearer
Stop worrying about others
And learn to put yourself first
So much you can discover
When you overlook the worst
Despite all the flaws
You're worth it all
There's a peace inside of you
And it's been there if only you knew

Time To Get Up

Girl, you cried your last hurting tear
It's time we fight and face all those fears
You wear so many emotions
But now it's time for coaching
You are so beautiful inside and out
Let me show you how to face those doubts
Lift your shoulders, raise that head, and hold it high
Wipe those tears and freshen your eyes
Put that skin on glow
And let that healthy hair flow
Speak with boldness and walk in confidence
It's time to get up

Thought I Knew You

I thought I had you all figured out
But it didn't take time without a doubt
You played your games
Now I'm left with shame
The guilt I feel
Is very much real
But the tears I shed
Come from my heart that bled
Said I love you 1 time too many
Now I'm here wondering was it really envy
I can't even sit and blame you
Because I should've saw all the clues
A new lesson learned
Another scar yet I was burned
It's so much I want to undue
Damn I really thought I knew you

The Little Voice

Sometimes you know right
But your actions lead you wrong
Most times you put up a fight
Because things went on too long
Why don't you do it today?
Is this how you really feel?
How is this going to matter anyway?
I'm just trying to keep it real
Maybe I should keep quiet
Because my words may sound like I'm lying
But you know how life works
You got mixed feelings running wild
So wild you try to calm them down
Yet they scream so loud
Looking for an escape to get out
Little do you know
It's all in your head

No One is Perfect

You look in the mirror and see so many flaws
Yet someone finds you worth it all
Many judge what you look like
And sometimes even what you been through
Yet you are very confused
Because No one is perfect
Yet they seem to forget
Life takes you fast
Like a roller coaster you can't control
And things you want to last
Are held back like parole
Sometimes we want what we want
And life gives us what we need
Either way appreciate the journey
Because you'll see that it's worth it
And that no one is perfect

2019

I never judged pain until We met
Doing that was something I really regret
It's like I was living my best life
Well, only Until 2019
Here I am now wishing it was all a dream
One text message followed by a phone call
Drowning in sorrows trying to forget it all
It's nothing I can do to change how I feel
Damn 2019 was a big ass ordeal
A piece of my heart had left me
How was I dealing, only true ones could see
I became numb to the world I once knew
Losing this piece left me with big trust issues
2019 really broke my heart
And left me feeling torn apart
I heal then I break
Yet people think that I'm okay
Things will never be the same
But despite it all an Angel I gained
Now all I have is history
Because 2019 ended our future memories
I miss you a lot
And I love you forever
I also miss that bright smile
So, keep visiting every once in a while
As I continue to face the reality between
Now and the year of twenty nineteen

Free Run

Sometimes I want to pack up my feelings
Bottle up my emotions
And run away

Sometimes I get to thinking
My mind is literally racing
Yet I have nothing to say

Sometimes my heart feels a way
I want to love
But my actions could show a bit of hate

Sometimes it's harder to say what I mean
So I write it down
And then I feel all better it seems

No Judgement Zone

We've all had our days
And you know the ones I mean
The ones that leave us feeling green
The ones we get judged for even after the fact
The ones we tend to endure and never look back
Still don't get it
Well, I guess I can go into detail
The ones where we finally get to exhale
So, here's how it goes
We meet a guy and unintentionally go blind
Blind to the fact that it begins to hide our smile
But makes its way back every once in a while
We lose sight of who we once were
Like our life before everything is all a blur
And now we no longer act the same
Because his actions nearly drove us insane
We become the enemy ready to attack
When in reality, we just want the old us back

No More Waiting

So many times I could've settled
But God wouldn't let me
So many times I felt cradled
And He was only protecting me
I often felt betrayed
Got through some things I should've never forgave
But looking back, yes that was my biggest mistake
I regret ever turning around
But even more hate for bringing myself down
There's no more waiting
It's my life I'm upgrading

Do You Mind?

I wanna say some things I never said
Go some places I don't wanna forget
And if you think it's gonna be a problem
Then I hope you have some ways to solve them

All I ask is
One simple question
Do you mind?

I wanna feel a love I never felt
Experience some things to make my heart melt
Can you show me real love and never leave?
Is this something you wish to achieve

All I ask is
One simple question
Do you mind?

I wanna make memories that last forever
I know it may sound a little bit clever
It's the storms I want us to weather
Baby I just want us together

So, tell me do you mind
Tell me do you mind
Do you really mind
Or am I just wasting my time

Hurt The Same

Each time was a different person
And, a different lesson
Lessons leaving me uncertain
And in some heavy aggression
How did I end up this way?
Because the hurt was always the same
Was it that I gave too much?
Or was it that I wasn't enough
Tell me what I gotta do
Is there something I gotta prove?
Because eventually I'll go insane
If I keep getting hurt the same way

Caution: Yellow tape

Rip to all the times I doubted self
Rip to all the people who left
My life was slowly fading away
Could barely tell what or who was here to stay
Until I expressed how I felt
It's like I played the cards I was dealt
Before noticing who I really was
Going with the flow just because
Time is running out
Nowhere to turn now
Endless missions
For pointless reminiscing
So long farewell for what you see
Because that's only the
Death of the old me

Part of the Plan

Did I mention
It was never my intentions
To leave you reminiscing
But to you I became nonexistent
There was a lack of attention
And you weren't really catching feelings
So, I had to regroup and do some healing
The real you was revealing
Because I guess you didn't want dealings
Not sure if I was no long appealing
Or if it wasn't me you were seeking
But you left my heart bleeding
I wish I could say I was dreaming
But your actions are so deceiving
So, as I sit here grieving
And doing all that I can
Just tell me one thing
Was this part of your plan?

Message

2 am and I can't sleep
Because my thoughts are very deep
So, I pull out the paper and pen
And here is where I begin
I wrote a message to you
About my feelings and the truth
Somehow, it's better this way
Because I say what I mean to say
The message I relay
Are often memories that replay
Not sure if you'll ever get this
Because I'm just reminiscing

Pain in my Soul

I never knew life would be this way
Wondering will the pain ever go away
Sometimes it's so hard to let go
Maybe I just need to be held close
Because the pain in my soul
Is starting to take a toll
And it's like I'm losing control
But again, it's hard to let go
My heart skips a beat
And when triggered I can barely breathe
Can someone tell me what this is?
Or am I being too serious?
My body gets sweaty
And then my breathing becomes heavy
It's the pain in my soul
That's got my life barely whole

Stay Here

You never know who's real or fake
Until they start to walk away
The people I always wanted to stay
Left me and no not for a break
Trying to make the best of what was
Difficult situations causing me to rise above
Whoever new should come along
I hope that they don't lead me on
I must know intentions real and clear
No matter what just stay right here

Wanna Believe You

It's a lot of things I want to believe
But trusting you something I never achieved
Because your actions portrayed
What your heart never gave
And your love was only a simple little game
I let you tear apart more of my heart
When it was already slightly shattered
Ripping away piece by piece as if it never mattered
How could you?
More importantly why should I?
It's crazy cause I wanna believe you
But that's definitely ova with
And so are my silent cries

No More Running

I've learned to embrace my pain
And told myself no more running away
I would completely shut down
Didn't matter who was around
I would drown my pain with alcohol
Just to live in the moment
Thinking this was really helping me
But in reality, it was draining to see
Avoiding your problems doesn't help
Just look in the mirror at yourself
You can see the pain in your eyes
It's a look of defeat that says you're tired
So, take it from me and listen
No more running away
The problem is here to stay
Until you finally address it
Your life will be very hectic
You become your own burden
Because the trauma is constantly hurting

At War with Emotions

My smile says I'm as happy as can be but
My actions show anger at an all-time high
"I can do anything" is the fearless mentality in me that never
dies
And the support of anything I do always catches me by
surprise
Sometimes I can't seem to open up, most call that pride
I battle with depression and anxiety
And I write to get it out of me
I know it sounds like a lot
I can promise you it's not
I'm just Stuck at war
With some emotion baring scars

Anxiety: You Will Not Defeat Me

You work me up get me all anxious
Have me walking back n forth pacing
Make my levels of thinking rise
Only time and meditation make it subside
Yet you think you won me over
All out of luck no four-leaf clover
I refuse to give up
Not that easy I won't quit
Anxiety has struck again
But not in this body I rebuke it
I take a walk and ease my mind
Or simply write to pass the time
You thought you had me yet once more
So now I'm here to kick down that door
Anxiety was the trigger
But my faith in God was bigger
What the devil thought was gone take me
Only had him impatiently waiting
Waiting for defeat to be on his side
Out of control acts ones I can't hide
Breathe in, breathe out
And just like that without a doubt
I am free to be me
No worries no stress
I'm back to my regular life
Living at my best

Promises

Don't make no promises you can't keep
Just be honest as you can be
Because 1 lie leads to another
Then your words begin to stutter
Just keep it real with me
Before our bond becomes discrete

My Brother's Keeper
Long Live Tricky Tre June 28, 1992- June 4, 2019

Everything I do
Is in the name of you
You give me strength
In my darkest times
Remind me to keep going
And stop the unnecessary crying
You show up on my tough days
Letting me know it will be okay
Guiding me through when I'm unable
And for that of course I'm very thankful
Forever my brother's keeper
That I will always be
"Tricky Tre" will always live in me
There is no time limit on my pain
But another Angel I did gain
Happy Heavenly Birthday Tricky Tre
From your one and only lil sis Nae
4eva on my heart 4eva in my mind
Hate our journey had to depart
But God said it was time...

Who Knew?

Nobody could understand me
Nobody noticed how I really felt
Deep down what seems to be
Was usually the reason my feelings melt
Too pride high to admit it
Being the strong one I was committed
But my pain ran over
Sometimes taking over my composure
I started wearing it on my face
The strong could no longer be embraced
It took quite some time
So, all by my lonesome
I wrote powerful lines
Onto the paper they read like an explosive
In those poems I released
But wasn't truly healed
Darker me was unleashed
And the real me was revealed

The Story Must Continue

Until next time I enjoyed doing this
Sometimes I sit and look back to reminisce
The memories, the joy, and fun we had
Damn I wish good things did last
Always making the best with time
Something we can't get back nor rewind
Sending so longs and farewells out
There is nothing to sit and cry about
Despite the pain and trouble
No more dwelling on the struggle
Because Inside I hold what I been through
But nevertheless, the story must continue

STAY CONNECTED:

 sales@soulwritingllc.org

 @thesoulwriterslegacy

 @SoulWriterrr

 Soul Writing Speaks

 @thesoulwriterslegacy

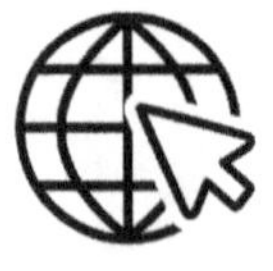 www.soulwritingllc.org

Other Books by the Author:

- Poetry: "It Comes from Within"
- Prayers: "You Are Not Alone"
- Journal: "The Recipe to Positivity"
- Poetry: "Expanding Your Horizons"
- Journal: "Stay Focused"